Activities for Elementary Physical Education and Recreation

JOHN SNIDER

authorHOUSE®

AuthorHouse™
1663 Liberty Drive
Bloomington, IN 47403
www.authorhouse.com
Phone: 1-800-839-8640

First published by AuthorHouse 4/21/2009

ISBN: 978-1-4389-5673-2 (sc)

Printed in the United States of America
Bloomington, Indiana

This book is printed on acid-free paper.

FOREWORD

Why do you want to teach physical education? Do you want to enhance the quality of people's lives? Do you want them to become productive members of the work force? Do you want children to develop all the physical abilities they possess? Do you want kids to realize the importance of leading an active life? Do you enjoy seeing kids in a moving environment?

If you answered yes to these questions, then you are on the right track to becoming a physical education teacher.

But, if you want to be a physical education teacher for merely these reasons; it's something to do until something better comes along; it's a good way to develop star athletes for the sports programs, then please find another career.

Also, you need to understand the shape of physical education today. School budgets and state tests are affecting it.

There is an old saying that goes "You don't appreciate your health until you lose it". A person's quality of life is defined most of the time by their health or lack of health.

Granted, there are times when birth defects, disease, and accidents have made achieving a healthy lifestyle impossible. But, not providing quality physical education classes in schools has immediate and far-reaching affects on the children.

Children who are fit achieve better test scores.[1] They also have better self-esteem and develop good attitudes toward the importance of maintaining healthy lifestyles. Children who are not fit or overweight do not possess the traits of those children who are fit. Children who are unfit are likely, later on, to have more medical problems, loss of work time, and shorter life spans.

How did we, as schools, get to where we are today. Today our school systems are **not** thinking about what we can do to insure that each child has the best opportunity to get fit and realize the importance of staying fit. Instead, our schools are trying to figure out what's the least we can get by with for physical education. More students per class, less physical education class time, and credit for physical activity outside of school are examples of what schools are doing to "just get by" in physical education.

Again, how did schools get to this point? One of the factors that have diminished the importance of physical education are the physical education teachers themselves. These

---

[1]   Study by California Schools

teachers had no purpose to their classes. There was no fitness achieved, no skills developed, and no understanding of the reason to maintain a healthy lifestyle. As a matter of fact, these physical education teachers did the same one or two activities everyday. This does not develop a respect for physical activity. Administrators who don't properly evaluate these programs have not helped this situation either. As an example, if a math teacher has trouble holding the attention of students or teaching any aspect of math, they are encouraged to seek help from their peers, school visits, workshops, and curriculum advisors.

This brings us to how we got to where we are today. Physical education is now being placed in direct competition with the academic or "test" driven subjects in our schools and physical education is losing this battle. Physical educators do not want a win. We just want a tie. Equal time. Equal support. Equal importance.

An administrator told me that until physical education has the same importance as the "tests" it will not receive the staffing, student-to-teacher ratio, or time needed to carry out a quality physical education class.

Money is the main issue. Schools are looking for programs to trim in order to save money. With its lack of importance, physical education is trimmed to the bare minimum or done away with totally (elementary). It is argued that elementary physical education is still provided but is taught by the classroom teacher. However, just because classroom teachers write physical education into their plans doesn't mean it's being taught. And it definitely is not quality physical education.

I find it interesting that the same people concerned with saving money or putting money into programs that are "test" driven will not even consider what they are getting or not getting for their money with respect to less physical education.

What good does it do to educate students and leave out the physical and healthy lifestyle education. What do we get? We get people who are affected with being overweight and obese. This causes diabetes, a high probability of them being absent from work, doctor's visits, hospitalization, and disabilities. Not only do these people become unable to **use** their education as productive workers, they also become a strain and drain on medical benefits and insurance rates. This affects everyone. So, are we getting a good return on the money invested in education? I don't think so.

The most disturbing thing about the issues of unhealthy lifestyles, sedentary living, obesity, and cutting physical education in schools is the report from the Center for Disease Control stating that this generation of school age children may be the first generation that doesn't outlive the previous generation for average longevity.

This is a crime. To have the technology, access to information, and ability to provide quality physical education in public schools and then **not** provide it is a crime.

What will bring about a change? What things need to occur to give physical education an important place in public schools?

Here's my list:

1. More money – Better funding by state

2. More separation between athletics and physical education

3. Don't treat physical education as a "feeder system" for athletic teams

4. Better teaching methods

5. Better evaluation of physical education teachers

6. Better teacher preparation by more colleges

7. More time for physical education in the elementary schools

8. Elementary physical education a minimum of 3 times per week

9. (NASPE recommends 150 min/week – 225 min/week for high school)

10. Required four years of physical education in high school

11. More opportunities for individual fitness development

12. Not using physical education as a punishment

13. (such as hold a child out of gym for not having their school work done)

14. Not changing gym schedules to fit programs or other

15. Develop state standards of achievement to be evaluated

16. More planning and evaluation time for elementary physical education

17. Better access to technology to help in the evaluation process

I'm sure there are other changes that could be added to the list. I'm sure that each of the items could be debated on the feasibility of it's making a difference. And, finally, the number one factor, money, would probably be where all discussion would take place and end.

Schools are run by making decisions on how to spend the money it has. State requirements and priorities determine these decisions. I feel the state and schools are setting requirements and affecting spending priorities with a short-sided, public relation-driven vision.

And remember that state and federal legislatures and school administrators were all, at one time or another, a student in an elementary and secondary school physical education program. Several probably remember physical education as being not worthwhile, boring, stressful, intimidating, or humiliating. It's no wonder that they seem to regard physical education as a program of low priority.

I've expressed my views on the shape of physical education in schools today to get your attention and hopefully to point out the importance of having quality physical education programs carried out by certified physical education teachers.

For you to become a physical educator who can develop a quality physical education program, you will need to acquire many skills and knowledge. Without the skills, knowledge and the commitment to quality physical education, you are just part of the problem rather than part of the solution.

Thanks for taking the time to read these thoughts on physical education and I hope the rest of this book will be helpful in your development as a physical education teacher.

CONTENTS

A ELEMENTARY PHYSICAL EDUCATION TEACHER

An elementary physical education teacher has to remember that he or she determines how good or bad their physical education program will be. The best activities ever will be wasted in any program being taught by a grumpy, mean spirited, super-sport wannabe.

But, a teacher who has the children's safety in mind, the children's growth and development in mind, and is fair and consistent with discipline will be on their way to having a great physical education program. Effective programs are taught by teachers who never stop trying to make the activities more fun, more beneficial for the students, and more relevant to the student's needs.

The following list contains my idea of teacher traits that are exhibited by effective elementary physical education teachers.

The teacher:

1. Has friendly demeanor.

2. Smiles.

3. Greets students by name (when possible).

4. Reads student body language and reacts accordingly.

5. States discipline policy in clear and simple terms.

6. Is consistent with discipline.

7. Always explains discipline in terms of student safety.

8. Explains proper dress for gym in terms of student safety.

9. Makes sure gym or activity area is safe.

10. Uses safe equipment in all games and activities.

11. Uses pre-class, during class, and post class routines that promote safety and good listening.

12. Always dresses appropriately for class.

13. Presents themselves in a professional manner during school, at meetings, conferences, etc.

14. Designs, develops and creates safe, fun and age appropriate activities.

15. Seeks new ideas!!!

16. Observes other school programs.

17. Attends workshops and conferences related to physical education.

18. Evaluates their own teaching, student performance, and activities.

19. Never feels that they know everything.

20. Passes along workable ideas to other physical education teachers.

CLASS MANAGEMENT

1. Expect correct "dress" for gym:

   a. rubber soled shoes

   b. no dangly earrings

   c. no dresses

   d. no sandals or shoes with no heel support

Note: Kids who forget, walk during class or participate in safe activities.

2. No one talks while I'm talking.

3. First offense during class – go to bleachers (short time). Second offense – <u>out</u>; sit on bleachers.

4. Make class so much fun that <u>no one</u> wants to be out.

   a. Use a variety of activities.

   b. Do not emphasize winning.

   c. Emphasize effort.

5. Explain on the first day of class that all of the rules are for the <u>safety</u> of the students.

6. Stress to each class that you are not mad at them if they have to go to the bleachers. They are to think about what they did and hopefully change it.

7. Be firm, fair, and consistent.

8. Use routines:

   a. Students entering class should know where to sit.

   b. Students leaving class should know where and how to leave.

MORE ON DISCIPLINE

The number one, big rule, in my class is no one talks when I'm talking. No one is bothering the person next to them. No one is messing with their shoes. Nothing! Your eyes are on me and you are listening to what I say and you're watching what I do. This is for your safety so you can learn how to throw, catch, pull, skip, kick, and everything else we do in gym. But mainly, you listen and pay attention for your safety and the safety of others. You can't learn, exercise, or have fun if you have blood running out of your ears.

If you are not listening when I'm talking or you talk when I'm talking, then I'm going to send you to the bleachers. Then, after a little bit, I'll let you come back on the floor. If you mess up again by talking when I'm talking, you go to the bleachers for the rest of that class. Two times and you're done for that day. I do not want you on this gym floor if you can't be safe. And, you can't be safe if you don't pay attention.

Now, if I send you to the bleachers, am I mad at you? NO! I'm never mad at you but if you don't listen or pay attention, then I'm going to sit you in the bleachers so you can think about listening better for your own safety.

Now, that big rule starts right now!

This little speech about the number one big rule in my class starts after I introduce myself to each class on the first day of school. I take roll call after the speech and I've sat kids in the bleachers before on the first day.

1. Think through all aspects of your rules.

2. Cut down number of rules – make it manageable.

3. Enforce rules – consistent, fair

4. Use safety as a basis for all rules.

Before the first day is over, I tell all my classes in grades one through four that today is the last that I will tell you to get quiet. I will wait for you to get quiet. And, when I'm waiting, you're wasting gym time.

You must be strict in your approach to this first day speech. But, temper it with light humor and comment that following rules and listening in gym class is important for their safety.

Be tougher at the beginning of school. It is easier to loosen up than it is to tighten up your discipline.

Try not to make the kids cry. Remember your big voice can scare them.

Don't allow tattle tales. This is a need for power thing and it disrupts class. Sometimes I send both the perpetrator and tattler to the bleachers and tell them to come back when they can get along.

We know to stay in close proximity to off task students but a stern quiet voice also works wonders.

If you expect certain behavior then wait for it or send the student who can't behave to the bleachers quickly.

Try to handle as much discipline in the gym as possible. However, send or take students to the principal if:

- fighting or hitting other students with fists

- knives, guns, etc.

- being totally and repeatedly disrespectful to you (teacher)

What if:

1. A student comes to class and wants to sit out because of injury for pain, then they want to come into class when something fun is going on? I don't allow them to pick and choose their activities. I make them sit and tell them "You're the one who chose to sit out". After the "fun" activity, ask them if they want to come back in. If they don't, start the fun activity again (if possible), but don't let them come in. It's all about who's going to be in charge.

2. A student just sits down on the floor and won't participate? Ask them to move off of the floor for their own safety. You may have to physically help them (nicely). Then make the activity fun. Exaggerate your praise for the performance of the students still on the floor. After class ask the non-participating student what the problem is. Sometimes you can also coax them back earlier, but give your attention, praise, etc. to the students doing the activity. <u>Your attention is for the kids doing work and cooperating.</u>

3. Students won't listen to directions? Use constructive fairy tales about what might happen if kids don't follow direction. For example, I told a class one time which direction we were going to jog and even moved this direction so they could see. When I told them to begin, the whole class went the direction I said except for one little boy who went the opposite way. He got halfway around the floor when he ran into a big, strong girl. The girl was not hurt, but the little boy flew back and banged his head on the floor. He ended up with ten stitches in his head and a broken nose. Now, whose fault was this? Right! The boy's fault. What did he not do? Right! He didn't listen. Now, be careful and pay attention for your safety!" (Make it believable, don't use names.)

4. A student does something good/praiseworthy? Give this student or students a

high-five, a hoop and holler. If you're going to tell them when they do wrong, you better tell them when they do right!!

5. Students are slow to respond to your directions? Learn students' names as soon as possible. Set time limit by saying "You have 14 seconds to safely put away the nerfs and sit on your number."

- Keep in mind that a combination of these discipline procedures can be used to fit other situations.

- Also, these procedures for techniques fit my personality. Everyone will need to modify most techniques that they learn about. Make them fit your personality, then your discipline will seem more believable and <u>sincere</u> to the students.

- Try not to back students or whole classes into a corner. Don't give them a "last chance" too early. But, if a student or class fails to behave with a last chance, then follow through with your discipline. There is no such thing as a last, last chance.

- A word about the "Bleachers". When I talk about sending students to the bleachers, I'm afraid that some might think that the students stay there for a long time. This is not true. The first time I send them that day is usually never longer than 1 or 1 ½ minutes and can be as short as 1 second. I send them to the bleachers to get their attention, to make them think about what they did wrong so they can safely participate. If they have to go a second time in one day, they are done for that class time if they are in grades 1-4. Kindergartners get more chances.

- Over the years, I've had some students that took "extra" effort to connect with. I've used techniques such as observing them at recess and talking with them away from the gym setting. These students took time to build a trust. Have patience and be observant.

Why is it important to have good discipline? Students who behave in physical education class are safer, learn more, get more done in a shorter amount of time, and are more cooperative.

Remember, a great lesson will go unlearned if the students are not paying attention or listening.

DISMISSING STUDENTS

Try to dismiss students in an orderly, quiet fashion. You want the last action of the class that day to be positive; not running, pushing, tattling, etc.

Here's the order of dismissing:

1. Say "sit on your numbers" (or squares)

2. Say "straightest, quietest"

3. Pick the straightest, quietest team or line to line up first

4. Position yourself close to the line to cut down on ditching, pushing, etc.

5. Dismiss the class

These are a few thoughts about discipline that I hope are helpful in managing an elementary physical education class.

Please keep in mind that the little people you deal with each day are not only looking to you for instruction, but also for guidance about how to behave in class.

Treat each student with respect.

CLASS ORGANIZATION

1. Numbers 1-8 in four (4) different colors form a square in the middle of the gym floor.

2. Each student in a class has their own number and the color of that number tells which team they are on.

3. Each team has its own triangle (same color). This allows a formation of four (4) relay lines in about eight (8) seconds.

4. Corresponding to the triangles are squares and X's are various distances on the floor. These give each team a specific spot to move to before they return to the line.

Example of Floor Markings

						R	e	d						
x Red	Red □			1	2	3	4	5	6	7	8			Δ Red
			8									1		
x White	White □		7									2		Δ White
		W	6									3	G	
		h	5									4	r	
		i	4									5	e	
x Green	Green □	t	3									6	e	Δ Green
		e	2									7	n	
x Blue	Blue □		1									8		Δ Blue
				8	7	6	5	4	3	2	1			
						B	l	u	e					

5. "Freeze" is the command that stops action at any time.

PAY ATTENTION!!

How many times have you heard teachers at all grade levels tell their class "pay attention" or "quiet" or "please get quiet"? Some teachers say these things twenty (20) to thirty (30) times a day. I do not have time for this. I tell my classes the first day I see them that I will not tell them to get quiet anymore the rest of the year. After the first day, I will wait until they are quiet and their eyes are on me before I start the day's activities. Students soon learn that there will be no fun or activity until they're quiet. I use this same technique when changing activities and before I give any directions during class.

I do not use this method with my kindergarten classes until January or February. There are always a few that cannot or will not get quiet. These students are set in the bleachers. They will get a second chance that day, but the next offense puts them in the bleacher for the rest of that class time.

Reward good listeners! Tell their teachers what a good job the class did. Give them high fives; whatever you feel is appropriate. Try to be consistent with this technique. Remember, listening and paying attention is a learned behavior.

- During activity, games, movement, students can make as much noise as they want.

FIRST WEEK

Intro & Warm Ups

Description: Students will sit along wall.

I will tell them my name and the one big rule which is "nobody talks when I'm talking".

Explain discipline procedure; sitting in bleachers, etc.

Take class roll.

Explain fire drill & tornado drill.

Kindergarten: practice moving and "freezing".

Grades 1-4: give students their numbers.

Talk about proper gym shoes, no dresses, safe jewelry, etc.

Warm Ups (K – 2)

skip, gallop, bear crawl, crab walk

Warm Ups (3 - 4)

push ups, sit ups, jumping jacks

Δ's – who sits out front, wait until person in front comes past ear before you go.

1ˢᵗ Plan	2ⁿᵈ Plan
Intro	Warm Ups
	K – moving, self & general space
	use parachute with K as an ice breaker
	Gr. 1-4 sit on Δ's and running
	Gr. 2-4 carioca

NOTES: Work on skipping with kindergarten.

Have kids help new 2-4 grade students with carioca.

Introduce carioca to first grade students next week.

ACTIVITIES

The next few pages consist of a <u>few</u> activities that my students enjoy. These activities, combined with our "old" standards of jumping rope, jogging, sprinting, long jumping, floor hockey, indoor baseball, New York City stickball, give the students a good workout and a chance to develop movement skills.

The activity descriptions are short and simple. I did not want the reader to think that there is only one way to do these activities. Change whatever you want to make these activities fit your program or style of teaching. That is what I've done over the years. I have gathered activity ideas from my college classes, observing other teacher's physical education classes, physical education books and videos, and from my own students.

My own students have shown me how we could change an activity to make it better and more fun. Sometimes I will ask them "How can we make this game (or activity) better?" Sometimes I'll get an idea by observing my class.

A good teacher has to be willing to experiment to make classes fun and beneficial for the students.

All of my classes (K-4) are able to do the following activities with some modifications to fit the grade level. You will need to observe your classes during these activities and make changes when needed.

DESCRIPTION OF ACTIVITIES

BUCKET BALL

Formation:

Two (2) to four (4) buckets (10 gallon).

Divide class in half.

Activity:

Each team must gather nerfs into their bucket using their feet.

   a.   soccer kicks, etc.

   b.   sits with ball between feet to lift it into bucket.

Two (2) to three (3) minute time limit for each game.

The more nerfs you use the better.

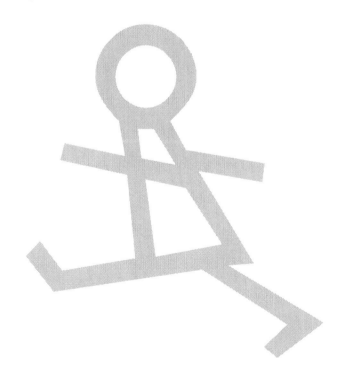

Buckets in the Air

Formation:

Attach rope over top of basketball backboards.

String buckets through the rope.

Leave a tail of rope so you can raise and lower rope.

Activity:

Toss and/or throw nerfs in buckets.

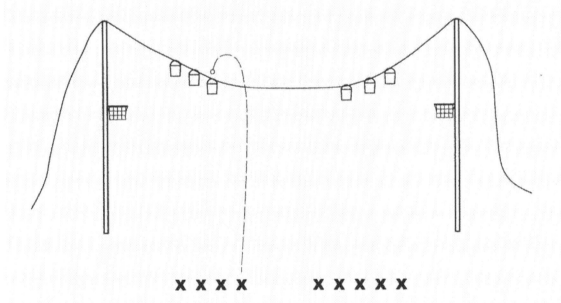

X X X X   X X X X X

ROPES AND SCOOTERS

Formation:

Attach to wall or have ropes held at each end by students.

Ropes should be the length of the width of the gym floor.

Seven (7) to nine (9) ropes work good.

Divide class into small groups.

Activity:

Students take turns pulling themselves the length of the rope on the scooters.

Variations:

pull while sitting

pull while kneeling

pull while lying on back

pull while lying on belly

Note: When going on back or belly, students with long hair should put their hair down the back of their shirt.

GYM SCOOTERS

Scooter Relay

a. class divided in four (4) lines.

b. students take turns on gym scooters.

c. students may go on belly (long hair down back of shirt), bottom, or knees.

Teacher can vary the distance that student rides.

Teacher can vary direction of ride.

□	□	□	□
Δ	Δ	Δ	Δ
X	X	X	X
X	X	X	X
X	X	X	X

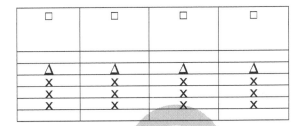

Caution:

Watch fingers (going under wheels)

Long hair goes down under the back of shirt

(so it doesn't get caught in wheels)

ROPES AND SCOOTERS

Formation:

Seven (7) or eight (8) ropes either tied across gym floor or held at each end by students while sitting on floor.

Activity:

Students use hands to pull themselves across the floor sitting, kneeling, laying on back or belly, while on the scooter board.

- Students may <u>not</u> stand on scooters.

- Try to use soft rope.

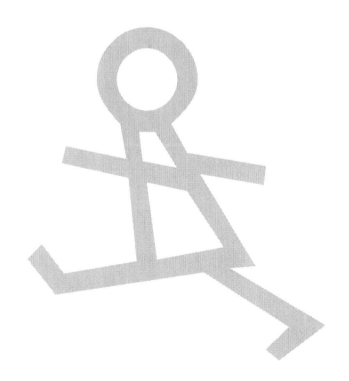

SCOOTER TOWN

Formation:

Use plastic floor tape or lines on basketball court to represent roads/streets.

Activity:

Students work in groups of two (2) or three (3) and take turns using gym scooters to explore the country, city, etc. on the roads.

Students may use sitting, knees and belly method of riding scooters.

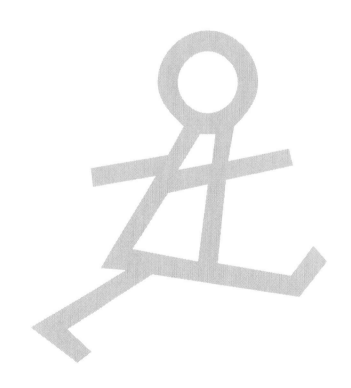

BEAN BAG CATCHING

Formation:

Self space – sitting, standing, kneeling, back

Activity:

Toss bean bag and catch with:

hands

scoops

frisbee

- Switch hands (right: left) and use both hands.

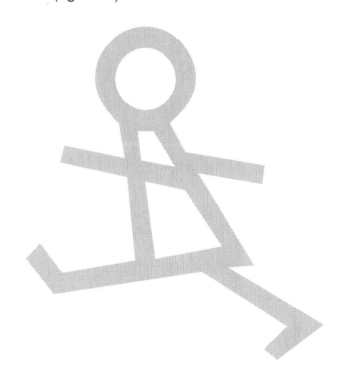

TWO STEP TOSS

Formation:

Partners facing each other through middle of floor from end to end.

Activity:

Partners stand and face each other with toes touching.

They both take two (2) steps back.

They toss a bean bag back and forth while counting their catches.

If they catch ten (10) in a row, they step back two (2) more steps each.

If they miss at anytime, they touch toes and start over.

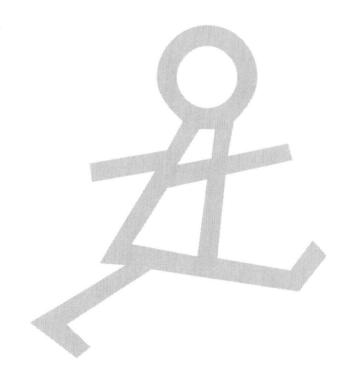

TEAM PIN TOSS

Formation:

Each team sits in a line equal distance from a row of styrofoam pins (or milk jugs, etc.)

Activity:

Teams take turns throwing a bean bag at pins until all pins are knocked down. (students throw, go get bean bag, bring it back to next person, go to end of line).

When all of pins are down, team puts bean bag in the middle of floor and then sits down in a straight line.

- This can be game – first team done wins.
- Students can throw overhand or underhand.

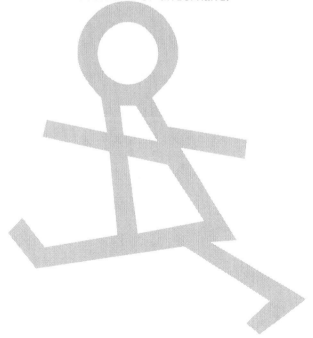

STANDING BRIDGE

Formation:

Four (4) or five (5) lines of students.

Activity:

Students in line, stand face forward, spread legs.

Last person in each line starts by crawling through legs of their teammates. When they crawl out the front, they stand and spread their legs.

Repeat with each last person and the bridge will <u>move</u>.

- Can be a race.

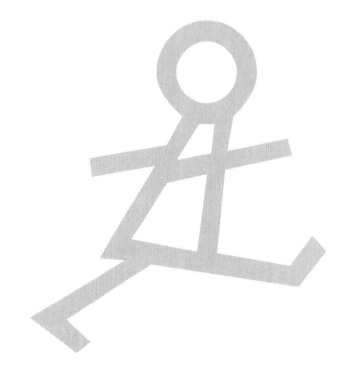

HULA HOOP HORSESHOES

Formation:

Two (2) rows of hoops spaced from one end of floor to other end.

Both rows 15 ft. apart (closer for K – 1).

One (1) person behind each hoop.

Activity:

Students toss two (2) bean bags at hoop across from them.

Student across from them is their opponent.

A toss inside the hoop is five (5) points.

A toss that ends up on top of hoop is five (5) points.

All other tosses are zero (0).

If a student catches a bean bag when it's tossed, it is five (5) points for the opponent.

- This game also works if you rotate the students one (1) hoop to the left every sixty (60) seconds. After each rotation, the new opponents start a new game with score at zero (0) to zero (0).

- After the rotation process is learned, the students can play in pairs with two (2) people playing two (2) people using four (4) bean bags.

UP THE LADDER - TOSSING

Formation:

Each student has a bean bag.

Each student stands on throwing spot in front of a bucket (10 gal.).

Nine (9) or ten (10) buckets are spaced along one side of the gym.

Throwing spots or tape is placed in front of each bucket. Distance depends on grade level.

Activity:

Each student tosses at bucket.

If bean bag goes in, student gets their bean bag and moves to the right (up ladder) one (1) bucket and takes a turn tossing.

If bean bag doesn't go in, student takes bean bag and goes to the left (down ladder) one (1) bucket and tries again.

Students try to get to the top of ladder.

If student makes toss in top bucket, they jog to bottom bucket and start up the ladder again.

Each student may have to wait for a turn when going up or down the ladder.

PIN BLAST

Formation:

Class divided in two (2) teams.

Each team stands behind a line (20-25 ft. apart) of ten (10) to fifteen (15) styrofoam or plastic pins.

Thirty (30) to forty (40) nerfs are spread out behind each line of students.

Activity:

Each team throws nerfs at other teams' pins.

Teacher can wait until all pins are down for one (1) team.

Teacher can use time limit for each game.

- If student accidentally knocks down their own pin, it stays down for duration of the game.

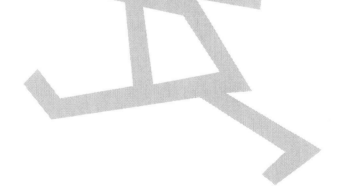

DUCKS AND RABBITS

Formation:

Class divided into two (2) teams.

Each team standing behind a throwing line.

The two (2) throwing lines are 20-25 ft. apart (like Pin Blast formation).

Thirty (30) to forty (40) nerf balls are spread out behind each line.

Activity:

Teacher rolls frisbee in the area of floor between the teams.

The students throw nerfs at these "Rabbits".

The teacher may also sail frisbee (vertically) between the lines and the students may throw at these "ducks".

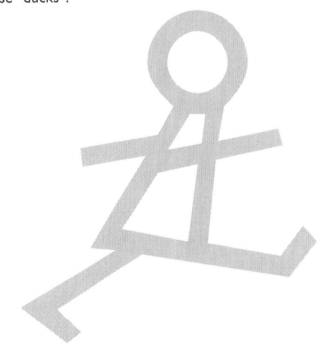

HUMAN FIELD GOALS

Formation:

Students with a partner.

Each pair of partners has one (1) styrofoam (soft) pin and they sit near a wall.

Activity:

One (1) partner faces wall (3 ft. away) with their arms up (goal post).

Other partner steps back five (5) steps from goal post, puts pin on floor, takes a two (2) step drop and tries to kick pin through the goal post.

Partners switch jobs after each kick.

If there is a group of three (3), two (2) people lock arms and raise opposite arms for goal post.

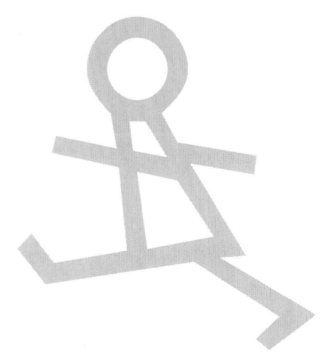

HUMAN MOP

Formation:

Students in groups of three (3).

Each group has one (1) firm plastic wand.

Each group spaced along same side of gym floor.

Activity:

Each group has one (1) person lay on back holding one (1) end of stick. The other two (2) in group grab stick toward other end.

The two (2) students standing pull (mop) the student on their back across the floor.

When group gets to other side of floor, they change person to mop and pull to the other side.

Each group repeats until everyone's had two (2) or three (3) chances to be the mop.

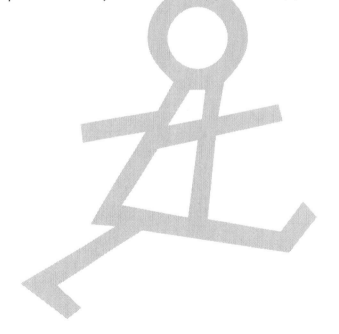

SNAKES AND STATUES

Formation:

Students in self space on belly.

Teacher standing with bag of nerf balls.

Activity:

Students crawl like snakes.

Teacher rolls or softly tosses nerfs at the "snakes".

If nerf touches "snake", the snake must stand and freeze like a statue.

The snakes can turn the statues back into snakes by touching the statues' shoes with their hands.

Teacher does not toss nerf toward the heads of "snakes". (They will duck their heads by reflex and they might bump their chins on the floor.)

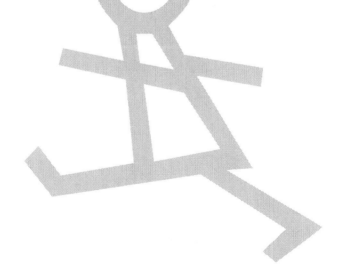

PUTT-PUTT GOLF

Formation:

Student with partner or groups of three (3).

Students share a styrofoam or rubber headed putter.

Putting course is laid out using styrofoam noodles as sides of "fairways" for each hole.

Plastic golf balls are safe.

Activity:

Students take turns with partners trying to putt ball in hole in the least amount of putts.

Teacher uses a time limit to switch groups from hole to hole.

Teacher sets "par" for each hole.

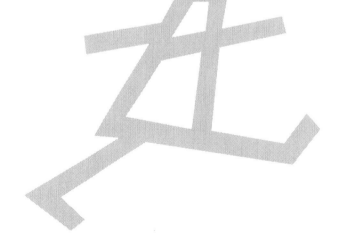

- Eight (8) to nine (9) different shaped "fairways" holds student's interest.

- Plastic putting cups will be needed – One (1) per hole.

MOLLY POLE

Formation:

Students standing in a circle.

Teacher stands in middle holding the molly pole.

Circle of students should be big enough that molly pole will just reach students' feet as teacher trails it on the floor.

Activity:

Teacher turns molly pole around circle.

Students jump pole as it passes.

If pole touches student, that student steps <u>back</u>, does ten (10) jumping jacks and returns to circle (while the teacher continues turning).

- Teacher make sure end of pole touches floor while turning and don't turn so fast as to trip students.
- Teacher may reverse direction of turn at any time.

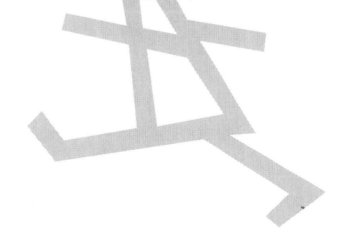

TROPHY FREEZE

Formation:

Students in self space lying on their belly.

Activity:

<u>Teacher blows whistle</u> – Students stand and freeze in a representation of any sport. This makes them look like the tops of sport trophies.

<u>Teacher blows whistle</u> – Students lay on belly and think of a sport to freeze in next.

<u>Teacher blows whistle</u> – Students freeze in different sport figure.

Repeat.

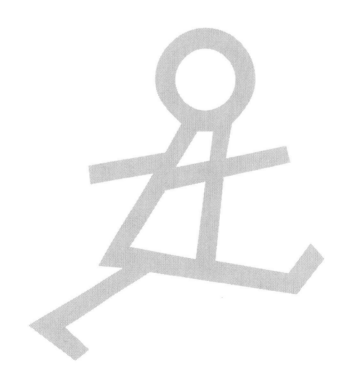

GOING TO THE BEACH

Formation:

All students standing on same side (out of bounds line) of floor.

Students should be arms length away from each other.

Activity:

Teacher says "Let's go to the beach!"

Students jog to other side line (without touching walls).

When all students have jogged to the beach, the teacher says "We forgot our _____ (blanket, radio, etc). Let's jog back home and get it.» When all students are at home, the teacher says «Let's go to the beach!»

And the process is repeated.

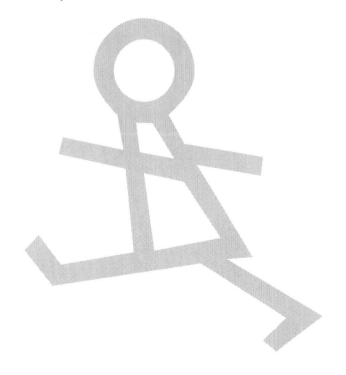

CROSS COURT HOCKEY

Formation:

Ten (10) to fifteen (15) pins set along each side of gym floor.

Four (4) or five (5) orange cones spaced out in middle of floor from end to end.

Half of the class on either side of line marked by orange cones.

Each student has floor hockey stick.

There are thirty (30) to forty (40) pucks spread out on floor.

Activity:

Each team hits (sweeps) pucks toward other team's pins.

Players may guard (goalie) their teams' pins.

Can use time limit for games or stop when all pins of one (1) team are knocked down.

CLEAN HOUSE HOCKEY

Formation:

Half of the class on each end of floor divided by center line.

Their half of floor is their house.

Each student has a floor hockey stick.

There are thirty (30) to forty (40) pucks spread all over the floor.

Activity:

The students use sticks to hit (sweep) the pucks (bugs) out of their house into the other team's house.

Best to use short (40 to 60 second) periods of cleaning.

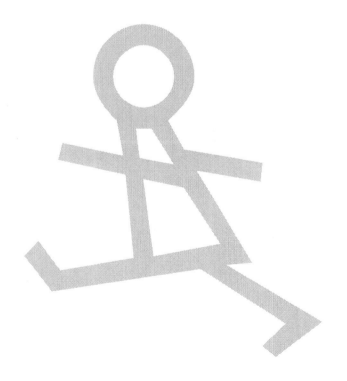

HUMAN BRIDGE

Formation:

Class in four (4) or five (5) lines.

Activity:

First person in each line makes a bridge by touching the floor with just their hands and feet.

Next person crawls under the bridge and makes another bridge next to the first.

Rest of team follows.

When all the team has gone under, the first person goes again and it starts all over.

The bridges will look like they are «moving» down the floor.

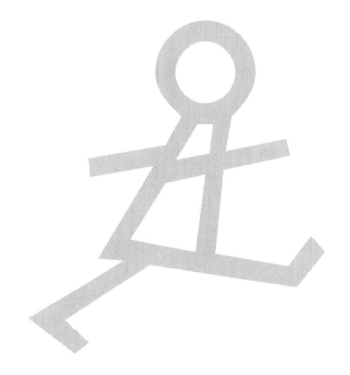

PARACHUTE #6 CHALLENGE

«Parachute Touch the Ceiling»

Formation:

Students hold parachute waist or knee high.

Activity:

Teacher says «pull up».

As students lift chute near chest level, teacher says «let it go».

If release by class is clean (together) the chute will rise up.

Point System	barely touch	1 point
	drags across	3 points
	sticks (jelly fish)	5 points

- Set specific time limit: 10-12 minutes
- Stress teamwork and organization.
- Classes compete against other classes.
- Make sure the chute will not catch on lights or ceiling.

PARACHUTE #5 CHALLENGE

Formation:

Students hold chute waist high near a basketball hoop.

Teacher places 24" beach ball on chute.

Activity:

Class lifts and pulls down chute, on command, making the ball "pop up".

Class can direct ball toward hoop by having students nearest the hoop hold chute "tight" to their waist and not lift up with the rest of class.

Set short period of time for this challenge. "Ball in the Hoop"

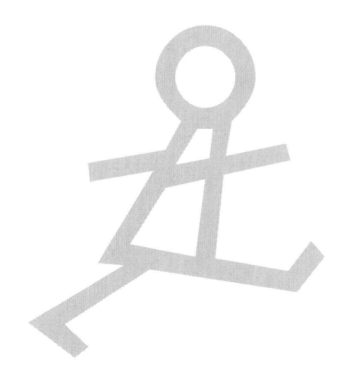

PARACHUTE #4

Formation:

Sit ups – students sit on floor and hold chute on their waist.

Activity:

Lean back and "touch chin" with chute

Sit up and "touch toes" with chute

Repeat a & b

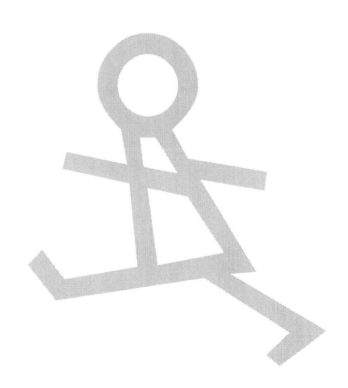

PARACHUTE #3

Barbershop

Formation:

Students take turns sitting under chute while class shakes chute then lifts it on teacher command.

Activity:

The static created by the chute will make most kids' hair stand up when the chute is lifted.

- Most classes will shake and lift the chute until their arms fall off in order to make others' hair stand up.

Club House

Formation:

Students lift up chute.

Students take one step forward.

Activity:

Students sit down while holding the chute on the floor behind them.

Students lean back and kick the top of chute (everyone under the chute at this time).

PARACHUTE #2 AIR BALL

Formation:

Students in circle with chute held near feet.

Teacher holds nerf or light weight ball near outside edge on the floor.

Activity:

Command – "pick it up" – students lift chute as high as possible.

Command – "pull it down" – students pull chute to floor hard.

Air from chute pushes ball along the floor.

You can vary distances, hit targets, etc.

Don't forget to talk about:

a. what makes ball move?

b. who supplies the power?

c. teamwork!

PARACHUTE #1

Formation:

Students in a circle – hold parachute waist high.

Activity:

<u>Shake</u> – small and big waves.

Pick it way up – pull it down – we call this the hair dryer.

Popcorn

Throw nerfs on chute. Students <u>shake</u> them off.

Rockets

With nerfs on chute students "on command" pick chute up – pull it down hard. Nerfs will fly up like a rocket.

Snake

Put jump ropes on chute. Students shake until "snake" goes in the hole or off chute.

Mouse Trap

Students make small, slow waves until little balls or nerfs go in hole of chute.

BALL HANDLING & DRIBBLING

1. Two (2) hand drop and catch

2. One (1) hand push down and catch

3. Wall pass – bounce and catch

4. Two (2) hand dribble

5. One (1) hand dribble

6. Dribble and walk

7. Dribble while moving without looking at the ball

8. Dribble around obstacles

9. Using right and left hands

10. Run and dribble

11. Dribble – run-stop-run-stop (keep dribbling)

    a. Roll ball with fingers around body

    b. Roll ball in and around feet – figure 8

    c. Figure 8 without letting ball touch floor

STUNTS AND TUMBLING

1. Forward Roll

    a. Sit like baseball catcher

    b. Hands flat on the floor

    c. Tuck chin

    d. Roll (try to keep arms "equally bent")

2. Backward Roll

    a. Sit like a baseball catcher – with back to the mat

    b. Hands clasped behind the head

    c. Roll back keeping knees close to the chest

    d. Throw feet into air imaginary bucket at the end of the mat

3. Activities

    a. Series of forward rolls (and back rolls)

    b. Pyramids – two (2) on the bottom only

Note:

   • Use mats

   • Keep it simple

   • May want to have back roll optional

   • Keep eye on students (necks)

   • Start kindergarten with log rolls to get used to mats

NFL FRISBEE

Formation:

Teacher has four (4) frisbees.

Activity:

Students take turns running to catch a frisbee thrown in the air.

- Teacher has to wait until floor is clear before throwing to student on the run.

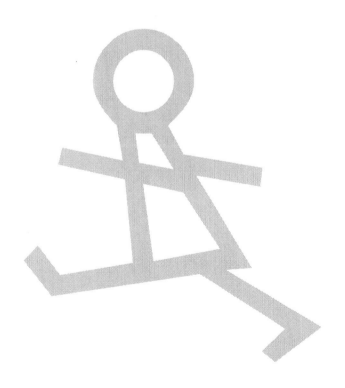

BEAN BAG CATCHING
(USING FRISBEES)

1. Equipment: One (1) bean bag and one (1) frisbee per student.

2. Use frisbee to catch bean bag

    a. alternate hands

    b. both hands (pancake flip)

    c. catch under legs

    d. catch while kneeling, standing, sitting, etc.

    e. catch behind back

    f. kick bag up with foot and then catch

3. Drop frisbee on floor and use it as a target to toss the bean bag on.

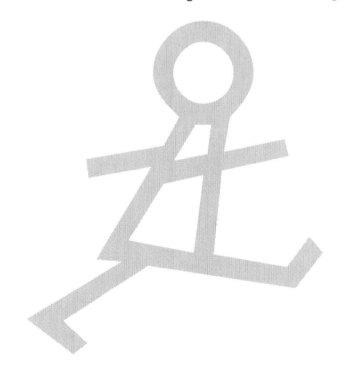

NUTS & BOLTS

Equipment:

One (1) set of 9/16 nut and 2" bolt (for each student).

Object:

Turn nut on and off each bolt using left and right hand.

Spin nut on and off using each hand.

Kindergarten, 1ˢᵗ grade activity – Good for small muscle manipulation. Carries over to writing skills.

NOTE: Make sure all nuts and bolts are returned at the end of class.

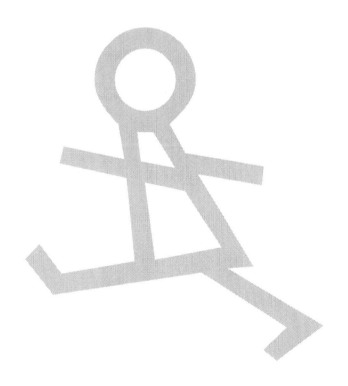

HULA HOOPS - TRICKS

1. Students try to roll hoops with back spiral:

   a. Use underhand toss with forward motion.

   b. Release the hoop while pulling down and back with a wrist snap.

2. Tricks to use when hoops roll back to students.

   Examples:

   a. Catch hoop with either hand or foot

   b. Catch hoop with neck

   c. Do front or back road

   d. Straddle jump over hoop

   e. Safely dive through hoop

   f. Bump hoop into the air with foot and catch hoop on the arm

NOTE: To get the idea or feel of making the hoop spin backwards, the student can put hoop over one arm and by using their dominant hand, pull the hoop down so it spins around arm. Then, using the same pull down, they can try to roll it with backspin.

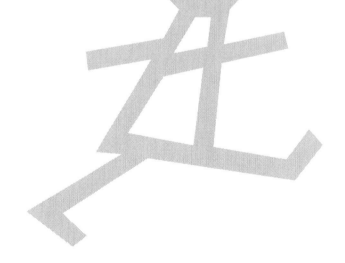

HULA HOOPS - CRAZY HOOPS

Formation:

Four (4) lines.

Enough hula hoops for every person on a team.

Activity:

Using one team at a time, teacher rolls hoop for each student to catch.

Roll hoop with back spiral.

Teacher calls out what to catch with:

> right hand
>
> left hand
>
> right foot
>
> left foot
>
> neck

Optional rolls:

Front road

> Student lays on back so hoop rolls over front.

Back road

> Vice versa of front road.

Bumble bees

> One student tries to catch as many hoops as they can when all are rolled at same time.

HULA HOOPS - MOVING THROUGH

Formation:

Students in four (4) lines.

Three (3) to six (6) hoops in front of each line.

Student given verbal or visual directions on how to "move through the hoops".

Activity:

Take turns until all in line are done.

When each team is done and sitting down, teacher gives each team another task.

Examples of movement:

Jumping in each hoop

Jumping in and out of each hoop

Running through

Bear crawl

Crab walk

One foot hop

Formations:

O	O	O	O
O	O	O	O
O	O	O	O
Δ	Δ	Δ	Δ
X	X	X	X
X	X	X	X
X	X	X	X
X	X	X	X

HULA HOOPS - GENERAL

Formation:

Students are allowed to hula hoop around their waist, neck and arms.

Activity:

They develop the feeling of the body, neck and arms being an object of which the hoop travels around.

Best way to teach – let kids experiment, watch you, and watch other kids, then try, try, try, try - - -!

NOTE: Make it fun – Don't embarrass them!

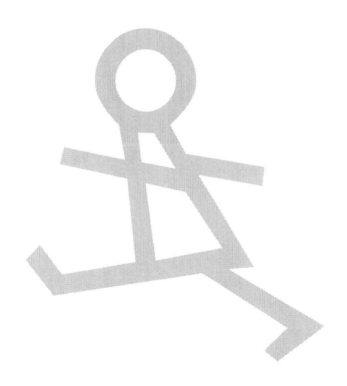

PARACHUTE CHALLENGE IN THE BASKET

Formation:

Students hold chute waist high.

Activity:

Teacher commands:

"Lift it up"

"Down" (to waist)

Teacher has placed beach ball (24" or less) on the parachute.

Action of class will cause ball to go in the air.

Class needs seven (7) people, with their backs to the basket, to hold chute tightly against their waist during the 'up' and 'down' action. This will cause the ball to travel in the direction of the basket.

NOTE: This is a hard activity. Need to set a time limit. Five (5) to ten (10) minutes.

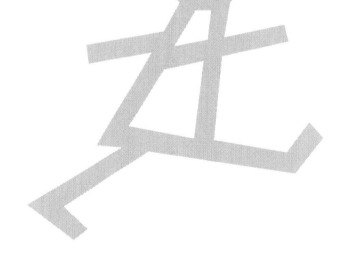

RUNNING FOR TIME

Formation:

Set a standard distance in gym for a running sprint.

Make sure there is enough distance for students to slow down and stop before the wall.

Class sits along wall (after warm-up).

Activity:

Teacher calls each student one at a time to run the sprint.

Teacher times and records each sprint.

Class then works on sprinting:

> running on balls of feet
>
> pumping arms
>
> head still and level
>
> fast and quick starts
>
> not slowing down on finish line

Re-time each student after one or two class times of sprint work.

NOTE: Object is to see if each student can beat their own time. Can let kids race after the second time run. Always inform kids that some people run faster against other people rather than time.

TOE-TO-TOE

Formation:

Class stands in a circle.

Class spreads feet until they touch neighbor's feet.

The legs should be at least shoulder width apart.

Activity:

Hit playground ball with hand only and try to get it to roll between someone's legs.

Students may use hands to block ball heading for their legs.

Pig:

If ball goes through legs once – get letter P

Twice – I

Third time – G

This spells PIG

Student with PIG goes in the middle and says "Oink-Oink" then returns to place with no letters.

CHINESE JUMP ROPES

Formation:

Try to get enough Chinese jump ropes (stretchy ropes) for a group of three (3) to four (4) students per rope.

Two students stand in ropes and act as holders.

Holders can use three (3) levels

    a.   around ankles

    b.   around calves

    c.   around knees

Activity:

Jumper tries to jump in and out with two (2) foot jumps, one (1) foot hops, etc., half turns and combination of all.

Each group switches jumper; holder on teacher command (whistle).

NOTE: Activity works best with music. Encourage creative (but safe) moves.

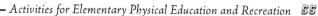

Jump Rope Challenge
(with big rope)

A.

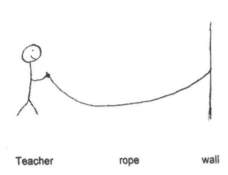

Teacher   rope   wall

1. Teacher turns big rope
2. Students jump till they miss
3. Class counts jumps

B. Four (4) or five (5) students at one time.

Group jumps until one misses.

* Teacher can try whole class at once if rope is big enough
or class is small.

JUMP ROPE VARIATIONS

1. Cross with rope

    a. Start by practicing arms crossing when they pass the head.

    b. Try to make elbows touch on the cross.

    c. Use wrist circles to keep the rope going.

2. Backwards cross

    a. Rope is turning from front to back.

    b. Arms cross but stay in front of body.

    c. Wrist circles allow the rope to travel over head.

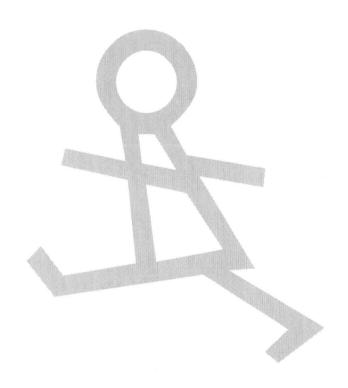

JUMP ROPE ACTIVITIES
STRAIGHT LINE

1. Each student has jump rope in self space.

2. Student lays rope on the floor in a straight line and then sits at one end of it.

3. Teacher demonstrates stunt – then teacher sits while students try the stunt two (2) times. When students are all sitting, then teacher demonstrates new stunt.

4. Examples:

   a. Jumping from side to side, down and back, the length of rope

   b. Bear crawl down and back

   c. Stand (straddle) middle of rope – Do four (4) half turns

   d. Straddle middle – Do two (2) full turns

   e. Older (grade 4-up) students can do examples a, b, c, and d in a routine (one after the other)

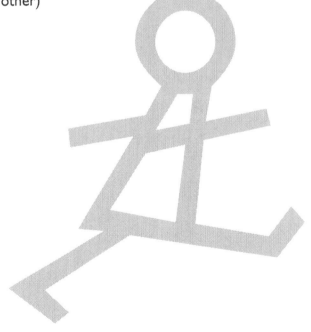

JUMP ROPE ACTIVITIES - CIRCLES

Formation:

Each student has a jump rope in a self space.

Student has made a circle with rope and is sitting inside.

Activity:

On whistle command, student will count number of times they can jump in and out of circle in ten seconds.

Students can:

    a. walk front ways on edge of rope

    b. walk backwards on edge of rope

    c. walk sideways on edge of rope

Students will try to lay their body on edge of rope.

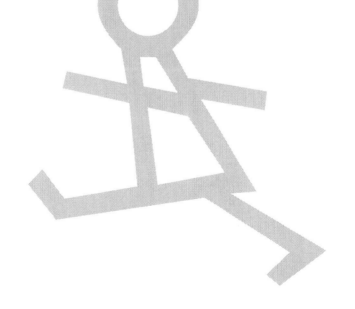

JUMP ROPE

Just beginning:

1. Students in self space holding jump rope <u>correctly</u> and facing teacher.

2. Teacher shows students how to swing rope over their head by using arm circles. Practice swing a few times.

3. Then swing rope over head and step over rope. Students may move at a walking pace around the gym.

4. Now students may swing and jump rope.

- After first few minutes of rope jumping, let kids rest (sit) and teacher shows students that jumping rope is a <u>two-part movement</u>;

     1. Swing first

     2. When rope hits floor – jump

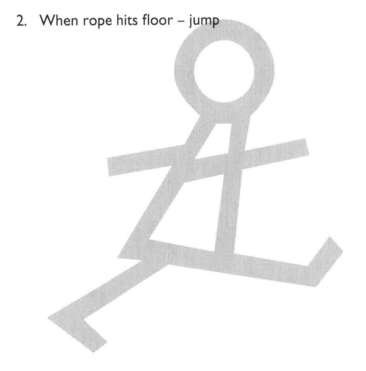

FRISBEE TAG

1. All students have 1 or 2 (if enough) frisbees to start each game.

2. There is no standing during games; students must crawl, crab walk, scoot on bottom, etc. to move around.

3. Object of game: slide (no throw) frisbee on floor to hit other people's shoes.

4. If frisbee touches shoe, the student must go to middle circle and sit.

5. Students in the middle circle can slide any frisbees that come near or in circle.

6. Students in circle are able to hit the shoes of students still in the game and get them out.

NOTE: Play each game 70 to 80 seconds. Don't usually play to one person left.

- Teacher shouts "New Game" to start everything over.

- Teacher calls "Up in the Air" – students sit holding frisbee up.

- Teacher calls "Ready – Go" to begin.

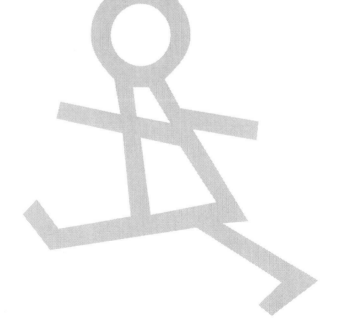

JUGGLING SCARF - #3

Formation:

Students in self space with two (2) scarves – one (1) in each hand.

Students are all facing same direction (toward teacher).

Activity:

Students <u>mirror</u> teacher's moves

Examples:

1. slide step
2. jumping jacks
3. arm circles
4. figure 8's with each hand

• Add music

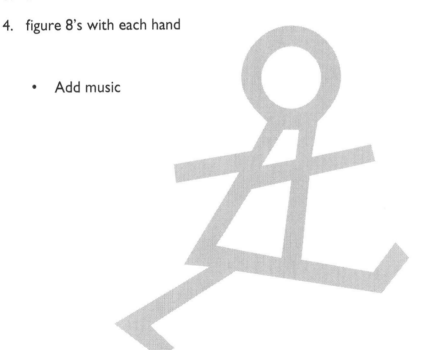

JUGGLING SCARF #2

Formation:

Students standing in self space with three (3) scarves each.

Activity:

Juggling three (3) scarves

- Find book on juggling for progressions

    cascade method

    crossover method

- Add Music

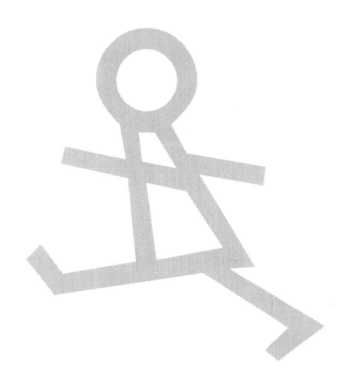

JUGGLING SCARF #1

Formation:

Students standing in self space with two (2) scarves each.

Activity:

They may toss and catch one (1) scarf – toss and catch both scarves with both hands – toss and catch both scarves using only one (1) hand.

- Add Music

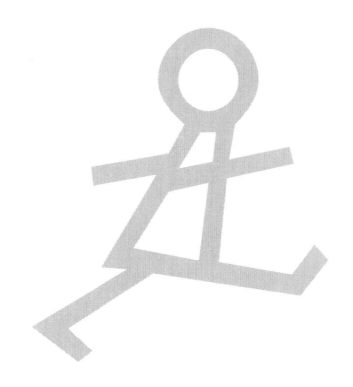

ROCKS & MULES

1. Need strong tug-of-war rope or strap.

2. Divide class in two (2) to three (3) groups.

3. Lay strap down the middle of floor.

4. <u>Rocks</u> (kids) lay on backs and grab rope or strap.

5. <u>Mules</u> (kids) stand and grab rope or strap.

6. Mules pull the rocks down the floor then switch roles and rocks become mules and pull rocks down floor to starting point.

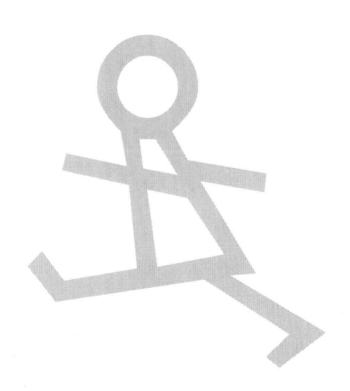

TUG-OF-WAR

1. Use strong tug-of-war strap or rope.

2. Divide class in two (2) to four (4) groups.

3. Divide by size of students.

4. Safety:

    Don't wrap rope around arms!

    Don't pull on rope when done!

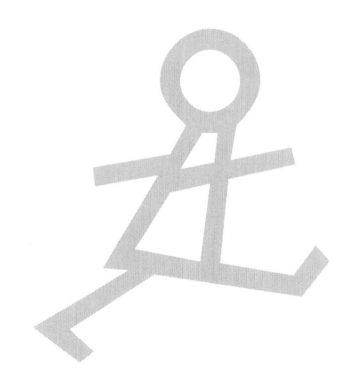

GIANT SCOOTERS

(also called Boat Races & Bobsled)

1. Class divided in two (2) to four (4) groups.

2. Construct giant scooter by putting enough regular scooter barrels under a tumbling mat or mats so the students can ride on them while others push or students riding push with feet.

3. Vary the distance of races.

4. The students who push and the students who ride should switch after each race or at the turn-a-round during a race.

NOTE: Can race group against group or each group against time.

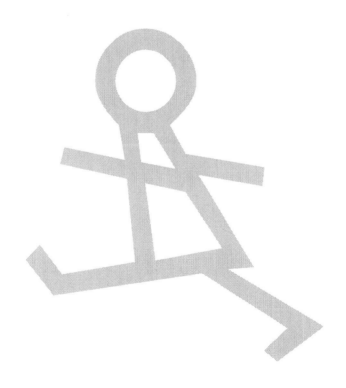

DYNA BANDS

1. One (1) medium-light pull band per student.

2. Stress safety – no snap, get plenty of room.

3. Do series of exercises to music.

Example:

Music – <u>40 Hour Week</u> by Alabama

Eight (8) pull downs

Eight (8) chest pulls

Eight (8) back scratchers - right

                                     - left

Eight (8) Hans & Fraun's

Eight (8) Bow & Arrow - right

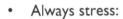

                           - left

- Always stress:

    Good posture

    Go slow

    Breath normal

NUMBER BALL

1. Equipment – Two (2) objects (ball, bean bags, etc.) to pass and retrieve.

2. Divide class in half with one half at each end of floor, standing shoulder to shoulder.

3. Give each team member a number with the head of the line being number one (1).

4. Teacher then calls a number:

   a. That #1 person from each team runs to center of floor and gets a ball.

   b. They each take ball to their own head of line.

   c. They go to end of the line.

   d. Rest of the team, meanwhile, is handing the ball down the line.

   e. When ball gets to the end the "called" number takes it back out to middle circle and lays it down.

   f. First team to get ball back to middle gets a point.

   g. Repeat process for all numbers.

NOTE:

- Ball or bean bag has to stay in middle circle or hoop or box.

- If object is dropped when passed, team just starts from where it was dropped.

- Object has to be passed to each team member without skipping; if not, no point.

Body Alphabet

Formation: Self Space

Activity: Teacher calls out the letters of the alphabet. Students shape their
Bodies to make the letters.

You can make your letters however you decide, but we make them like this:

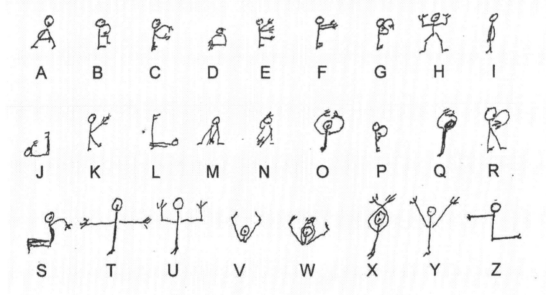

Can make this activity more fitness oriented by having students go to their
belly after each letter. We call this alphabet grass drills.

HOOP DROP

Formation:

Students in self space with a hula hoop.

Activity:

Each student holds their hula hoop with both hands over their head.

Teacher says "drop it" – students drop the hoop down over their body.

Then they jump out of the hoop with both feet.

Then they jump back in with both feet.

Then they pick the hoop back up over their head.

Repeat on command.

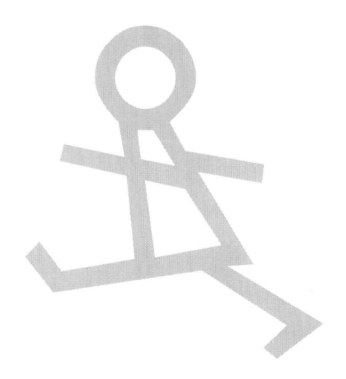

TROPHY TOPS

Formation:

Students in self space lying on belly.

Activity:

Students think of a sport while lying on belly.

On teacher signal, students stand up and freeze the action of a sport like the top of a trophy.

On teacher signal, students lay on belly and think of a different sport for their trophy top.

Teacher repeats with no more than three seconds of belly time.

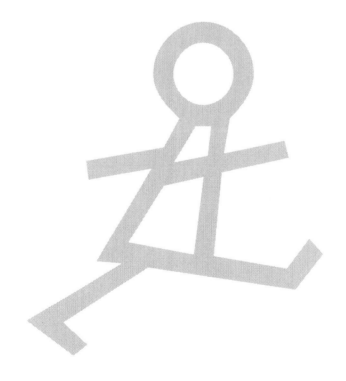

SIT AND SPIN

Formation:

Students in self space sitting on the Frisbee.

Activity:

Students use feet or feet & hands to scoot bottoms on Frisbee.

Students can also spin in circles while sitting on Frisbee.

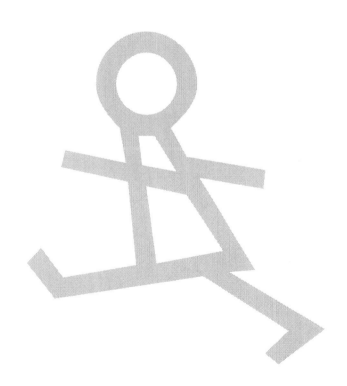

CONE TIPPERS

Formation:

Divide class in half. (Easiest – boys & girls)

Everyone standing in self space.

Twenty (20) or more orange cones sitting upright on floor (spaced out).

Activity:

On whistle, girls job; knock down any cone that's standing boys job; set up any cone that's lying down.

Stop on whistle signal.

Repeat with jobs switched.

- Caution students to watch where they move.
- Space cones away from walls.

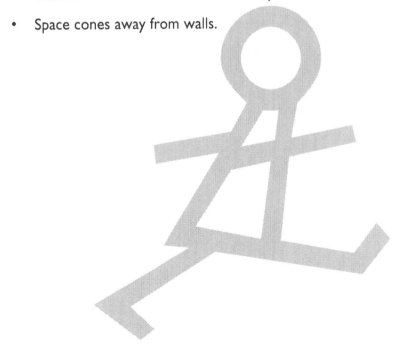

TEN - TEN - TEN

Formation:

Students standing in self space with a bean bag.

Activity:

Students toss & catch bean bag.

Standing:

   10 times right hand

   10 times left hand

   10 times both hands

Kneeling:

   10 times right hand

   10 times left hand

   10 times both hands

On Backs:

   10 times right hand

   10 times left hand

   10 times both hands

TICKET RELAY

Formation:

Four (4) lines

Activity:

First person in each line has a bean bag (ticket).

First person run with the ticket to a teacher determined spot and returns to their line handing the ticket to the next person.

Repeat until each person in line has a turn.

- Good way to teach relays.

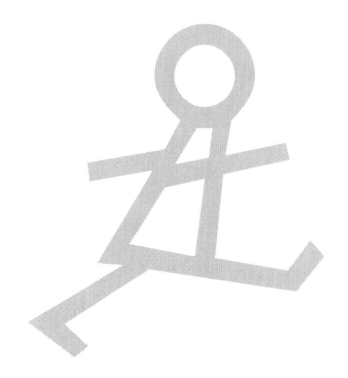

SWITCH-EM

Formation:

Four (4) lines

Activity:

First person in each line has a bean bag.

Another bean bag is on the floor out in front of each line.

First person runs to the bean bag on the floor and switches the bean bag they are carrying with the bean bag on the floor.

First person then runs back to their line and hands bean bag to the next person in line.

Variation:

Teacher can add bean bags so students have more switches.

- Use spots or markings on the floor so switched bean bags are kept in orderly line.

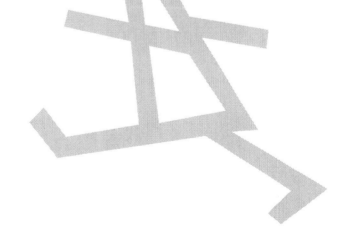

NERF ROCKETS

Formation:

Students in self space. Nerfs all over the floor.

Activity:

Students throw nerfs straight down to floor.

They see how high nerf will go after it hits floor.

NOTE: Coated nerfs with high to medium bounce are best to use.

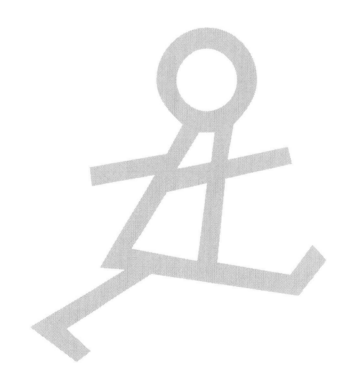

HULA HOOP DANCING

Formation:

Students in self space holding hula hoops like a dance partner.

Activity:

Play music. Students use slide step/or carioca.

Teacher leads the group (you and your hoop)

Can also spin your hoop (partner). Do-si-do.

Whatever you can think of that is safe.

It is also possible to do the electric slide with your hula hoop partner.

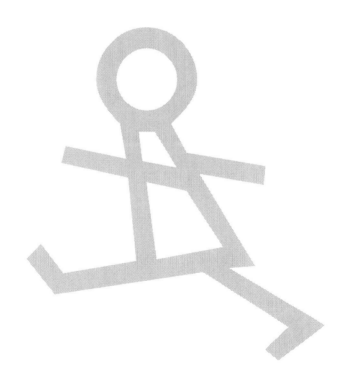

WALL SMACKERS

Formation:

Students in a self space. Teacher stands next to wall mats with a plastic wand in each hand.

Activity:

a. Teacher lightly taps wall – students walk to the beat.

b. Teacher hits wall with tap-tap-tap, tap-tap rhythm and the students skip.

c. Teacher hits the wall as hard as he/she can with both sticks – students jump as high as they can.

• Repeat

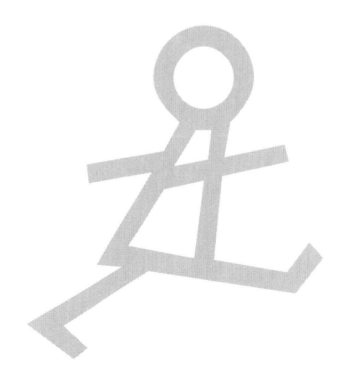

BOAT RACES

Formation:

Students lay on backs with feet facing side wall.

Activity:

Students use their feet (on the floor) to push their bodies across the floor (on their backs).

NOTE: Stop the race before first student gets to opposite wall. If students are sweating, they won't slide very well on the floor.

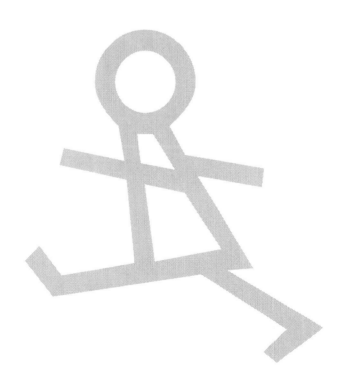

MUMMY HOOPS

Formation:

Students in self space. Each student has one foot in their own hula hoop. Nerfs are all over the floor.

Activity:

Students pull the hoop with their foot (mummy walk). They put nerfs in their hoops as they move.

Can see how many nerfs they collect in a certain amount of time.

Can take nerfs from other people's hoops.

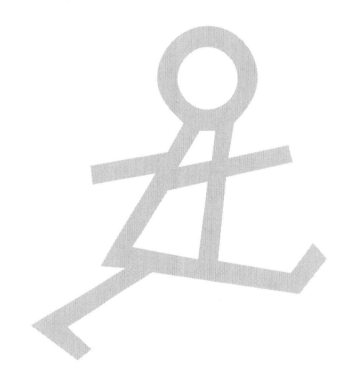

STEPPING STONES

Formation:

Students standing beside each other on side line of gym floor.

Each student has three (3) bean bags or three (3) poly spots.

Activity:

Students try to get to the other side of the floor by using their bean bags as stepping stones.

If they lose balance and touch floor with foot or hands, then they must start over.

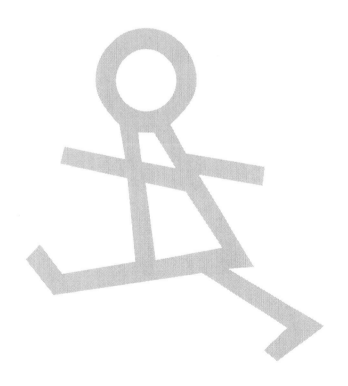

STEPPING STONES IN THE RAIN

Formation:

Same as stepping stones plus teacher stands behind students with nerf balls.

Activity:

Students try to get to other side of floor using bean bags as stepping stones while teacher lofts (lobs) nerfs in the air above students.

If students lose balance and touch floor with foot or a hand, then they must start over.

If a rain drop (nerf) touches student, then they must start over.

If student makes it to the other side of the floor, then they can help the teacher toss rain drops (nerfs).

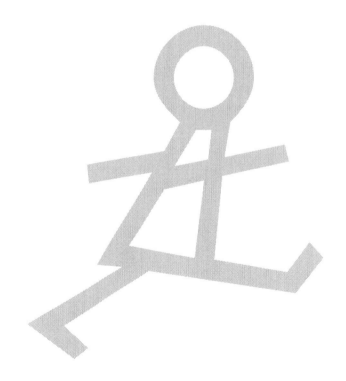

ADAPTIVE PHYSICAL EDUCATION

Think of safety first when adapting activities for students with special needs. After the safety aspects, comes how to make all (if possible) activities accessible and meaningful for the students.

Try to think of how you would participate if you had the same limitations. For example, put yourself in a chair when thinking about activity modifications for students in wheelchairs. Find out what a student with ADD is interested in and use that interest to help them focus during activities.

Remember to observe the students with special needs during your activities because your modifications will usually need further changing.

Finally, create a supportive class atmosphere by encouraging the class to acknowledge everyone's effort during activities.

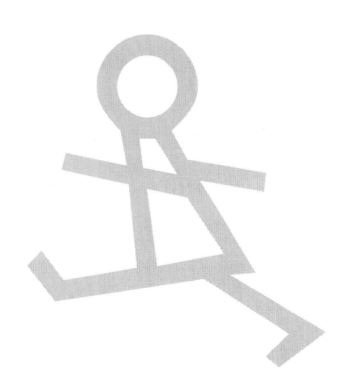

LAST BUT NOT LEAST

Hopefully, you will be able to use a few things from this book to help you become a good physical education teacher with a quality program.

Remember, ideas for activities, discipline, management, and organization, are **gathered, and not delivered**. Workshops, visiting other school programs and physical education websites are all examples of where you might find useful ideas.

And lastly, please keep in mind the **main reason** you are becoming a physical education teacher who wants to be a caring individual that creates a safe and positive environment. That main reason is the students.

DATE DUE

Made in the USA